DEPRESSION

The Real Cause May be Your Body.

Holly Fourchalk, PhD, DNM®

CHOICES UNLIMITED
FOR
HEALTH & WELLNESS

Choices Unlimited for Health & Wellness
Dr. Holly Fourchalk, Ph.D., DNM®, RHT, HT

Tel: 604.764.5203
Fax: 604.465.7964

Website: www.choicesunlimited.ca
E-mail: holly@choicesunlimited.ca

Editing, Interior Design and Cover Design: Wendy Dew-
ar Hughes, Summer Bay Press

ISBN: 978-0-9868775-9-9
Digital ISBN: 978-1-927626-00-9

To my Parents

For all their support and encouragement
My Dad for his ever listening ear
My mother for her open mind

IS DEPRESSION IN YOUR HEAD?

CONTENTS

INDEX

ONE

What is Depression?

Depression - what really is it? What really causes it? And what are the REAL treatments for it?

Our society has been horrifically misled regarding the subject of depression over the past several decades. While the experience of depression can be real and overwhelming, people can experience a wide spectrum of manifestations of it.

Did you know, for example, that there are many well recognized causes of depression that are physiological? Consider these possibilities.

Nutritional deficiencies that include:

- Omega 3s
- Glutathione
- B Vitamins
- Magnesium

Compromised organs:

* Gut
* Liver
* Adrenals
* Thyroid

Problems in any one of these, or any combination of these, can result in depression as the number one symptom.

So why is everyone who claims that they are experiencing depression either:

> put on anti-depressants (that the researchers know don't solve the problem)?

Or:

> sent to psychologists (who make the assumption that if the family physician hasn't identified anything else then it must be psychological when the family physician has no idea of all the different causes of depression)?

We are going to explore all the possible causes of depression in this little book so that you have a better understanding not only of what may be contributing to your experience but also what options you can consider to effectively resolve it.

STATISTICS

Health Canada statistics reveal that between 13-14 million people will experience a depressive disorder in any given year and that only about 20% receive adequate treatment.

Approximately 8% of the population will suffer from depression at some point in their lives and about 5% in a given year.

See:
http://www.bayridgetreatmentcenter.com/facts_statistics.html

The US claims that 18.8 million or about 9.5% of the US population, aged 18 and older, suffer from a mood disorder including:

- major depressive disorder
- dysthymic disorder
- bipolar disorder.

The most shocking statistic is that preschoolers are the fastest growing market for anti-depressants! There is something seriously wrong with this picture.

See:
http://www.upliftprogram.com/depression_stats.html

Centers for Disease Control and Prevention (CDC) claims that one in ten adults in the U.S. reports depression. They also found that the following were more likely to meet the criterion for major depression:

- persons 45-64 years of age
- women
- blacks, Hispanics, non-Hispanic persons of other races or multiple races
- persons with less than a high school education
- those previously married
- individuals unable to work or unemployed
- persons without health insurance coverage

See:
http://www.cdc.gov/Features/dsDepression

Many will call themselves depressed but don't fit a given criterion whether it is put forth by DSM (Diagnostic & Statistical Manual of Mental Disorders – published by the American Psychiatric Association) or ISD (International Statistical Classification of Diseases and Related Health Problems – published by the World Health Organization) or some other medical body. Many physicians and psychiatrists hand out prescriptions for anti-depressant medications on a regular basis without understanding the science behind what they do.

We are going to look at the following:

- What really is depression?
- What are all the different causes of depression – physiological and psychological?
- Understanding what your mind-body dynamic is doing and what you can do to resolve the issue.

Depressive Experiences

First, let's briefly look at all the different kinds of experiences that one can have that just get "dumped" into that one big bag called depression.

- One can have off days, and feel low – is that depression?
- Is it when you are tired and emotional and prone to crying?
- Is it when you are feeling "sad and depressed" because you lost a loved one?
- Is it when a relationship broke up and

you simply do not know what to do with yourself?

- Is it when your life is not where you thought it should be and you feel stuck?

- Is it when you feel hopeless and do not believe that there is light at the end of the tunnel?

- Is it that you go to bed exhausted and wake up exhausted and simply cannot get going?

- Is it when you have no interest in life and would rather simply roll over and forget the world?

- Is it when life becomes too difficult to manage because you cannot seem to think straight, make decisions, or concentrate?

- Is it when you are tired but when you go to bed you simply lie there and cannot go to sleep and your mind will just not give you a break?

- Or is it when you have no self-esteem, self-confidence, and do not believe you are of any value?

How many different experiences of depression are there?

You may have experienced one or more of the above at any given time in your life. You may have experienced it for a short period of time; for a long period of time; or it may come and go. You may even feel that it has always been there at some level.

What are the current recognized treatments for depression?

The World Health Organization (WHO) claims that depression affects about 121 million people worldwide and is the leading cause of disability worldwide. The WHO also claims that it can be treated but fewer than 25% of people affected have access to effective treatments.

But what is considered "effective treatment"? Some swear by their anti-depressant medications. Yet low serotonin has never been proven to be the cause of depression. Several years ago, the medications used to keep serotonin levels up in the brain were combined with medications to keep norepinephrine up in the brain as well. Now they even combine these medications with medications used to regulate dopamine levels as well. (These are the drugs used for schizophrenia.)

Why do these pharmaceutical changes keep happening when many of the actual researchers claim that it has never been proven that a chemical imbalance in the brain even causes depression?

Did you realize that it has never been proven that low serotonin causes depression? Even when low serotonin levels are correlated with depression, research indicates that there are variables that may be causing it.

See:
http://onlinelibrary.wiley.com/doi/10.1002/mds.870030308/abstract

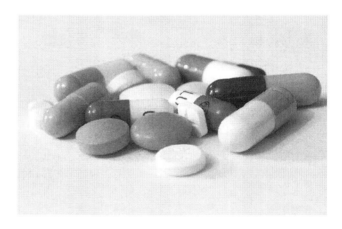

Further, there are way too many studies indicating that other issues are at play. Wikipedia even claims that Intensive investigation has failed to find convincing evidence of a primary dysfunction of a specific monoamine system in patients with major depressive disorders. Experiments with pharmacological agents that cause depletion of monoamines have shown that this depletion does not cause depression in healthy people nor does it worsen the symptoms in depressed patients.

See:
http://en.wikipedia.org/wiki/Biology_of_dep ression

Or we can look at what Dr. Mercola claimed in the following ...

(http://articles.mercola.com/sites/articles/arc hive/2011/04/06/frightening-story-behind-the-drug-companies-creation-of-medical-lobotomies.aspx)

Investigations were done to see whether or not depressed people actually had lower serotonin levels, and in 1983 the National Institute of Mental Health (NIMH) concluded that, "There is no evidence that there is anything wrong in the serotonergic system of depressed patients."

The serotonin theory is simply not a scientific statement. It's a botched theory — a hypothesis that was proven incorrect.

Or how about Dr Josephy Coyle, a professor of neuroscience at Harvard Medical School. "Chemical imbalance is sort of last-century thinking. It's much more complicated than that...It's a really outmoded way of thinking."

See:
http://www.npr.org/blogs/health/2012/01/
23/145525853/when-it-comes-to-depression-
serotonin-isnt-the-whole-story

Then if we go to the end of the paragraph...and so has no apparent effect.

We can add in here...but conversely, the gut contains 100 million neurons (more than the spinal cord) that connect with the neurotransmitters in the gut, i.e., serotonin, dopamine, and norephinephrine amongst others. What if would focused on a healthy gut rather than the neurotransmitters in the head?

Did you know that there is no way to identify the serotonin levels in the brain or that 90-95% of your serotonin is made in your gut (depending on the research that you read)? The serotonin made in the gut does not pass the blood-brain barrier to get into the brain and so has no apparent effect.

Did you know that a compromised liver, compromised thyroid, compromised adrenals and leaky gut syndrome all have depression as a major symptom?

Did you know that deficiencies in amino acids,

fatty acids, B vitamins, glutathione and anti-oxidants all have depression as a major symptom?

Did you know that our food is hugely deficient in the nutrients to make fatty acids, B vitamins, glutathione and anti-oxidants?

Did you know that the pesticides, herbicides, growth hormones, etc. in our food cause compromised organ functions, starting with the gastrointestinal tract (GIT) or our gut?

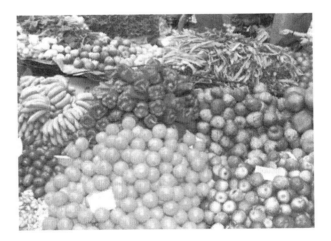

Don't feel alarmed if you did not know this:

- Most physicians are not taught these basics.

- Scientists and researchers are always amazed at how far behind the evidence the practicing physicians are in their knowledge.

- Pharmaceutical and pathology books are still producing the information that was believed some 20 years ago, so how do physicians stay up to date?

- When editors do not publish articles that challenge current thinking or the current protocols then physicians are at their mercy unless they are willing to take the initiative themselves to stay current with new research findings.

For your information, physicians require six CE (Continuing Education credits) per year. If they attend the classes presented by the pharmaceutical companies, their expenses are generally paid, often in full. This is not to fault the physicians but why would they not attend these sessions when they and their families may enjoy wonderful vacations to exotic places paid for with the pharmaceutical companies' dollars?

However, if a physician chooses to get CE credits from anywhere else they must shoulder the expense. If you were the doctor, which would you be more likely to choose?

TWO

Who Diagnoses Depression?

The diagnosis of depression presents an interesting paradox. Who actually diagnoses depression in a patient?

Historically, it was either a psychologist or a psychiatrist. The psychologist will have spent twelve years studying psychology and have an understanding of the experimental design of subjective and objective testing, validity studies, reliability studies, and more.

Psychologists get a lot of training on how to assess different types of depression, both subjectively and objectively. Psychologists work with the patient's perception, interpretation and response to the external and internal world. These factors can have a huge impact on issues like depression, assuming depression is starting in the head with your interpretation and response to the world.

The psychiatrist, who had four years of medical school and then a residency for another four to five years with training in diagnosis, psychopharmacology, medical care issues and psychotherapies. The curriculum is usually governed by pharmaceutical companies. After a one year internship, a psychiatrist is allowed to diagnose depression and prescribe medication for it. As we will see below, these medications typically cause more problems than they solve.

The time came when the family physician was permitted to diagnose and prescribe medication for depression. They did this with no training on diet and the psyche or how these factors affect the mind. Rather, most of the training comes from the pharmaceutical companies and is primarily about how to manage symptoms.

So who really understands what is going on?

The psychologist has to take the word of the psychiatrist or the family physician that they have eliminated all other possible physiological causes, but as mentioned above, neither the family physician, nor the psychiatrist nor the psychologist, for that matter, has studied how diet or deficiencies in fatty acids, amino acids, glutathione, anti-oxidants, etc. can be the cause of depression.

Most of these professionals have apparently never studied or assessed how a compromised liver, adrenal fatigue, leaky gut syndrome, or a host of other physiological factors can cause depression. For knowledge on these matters, the patient must seek help from an alternative physician.

Note: In allopathic medicine your MD is taught to manage symptoms. (The alternative medicine practitioner is taught to eliminate the problem.) The problem with this system is that there is a conflict. If we simply manage symptoms with prescriptions we keep the drug companies well supplied with good profits but if we eliminate the problem, well, there go the huge profit margins. Someone has a massive vested interest in treating only your symptoms rather than getting you well. That is why billions of dollars are made per day on antidepressants!

Let's read what a few organizations have to say:

The Citizens Commission on Human Rights International (CCHR) claim:

1) Psychiatric drugs are big business and the psychiatric pharmaceutical industry is making a killing—$84 billion per year.
http://www.cchrint.org/psychiatric-disorders/

2) There are no tests in existence that can prove

mental disorders are medical conditions. Psychiatric diagnosis is based solely on opinion.

3) Yes, people can get depressed, sad, and anxious and even act psychotic. That doesn't make them mentally "diseased."

4) The campaign to "STOP THE STIGMA OF MENTAL ILLNESS" is brought to you by "Big Pharma".

5) Why Psychiatric labels are the problem.

Michael G. Conner, Psy.D. wrote: "Why do health care professionals in the U.S. recommend antidepressants without requiring more healthy and proven approaches first?" (He claims) There are two reasons.

1. Antidepressants are big business. (Are you aware that Americans spend more than 86 billion dollars a year on antidepressants alone, never mind all the other pharmaceuticals? Or, did you know that pharmaceutical companies spend nearly 10 billion dollars each year just on marketing and promotion? Antidepressants are one of the most commonly prescribed drugs and one of the most profitable drugs in America.

(In contrast, how much money is spent in the U.S. to promote awareness of healthier alternatives among health care professionals? This is not referring to simply the field of anti-depressants but applies right across the board.)

2. Marketing research reveals that people in the U.S. seem to believe drug marketing. Despite the increasing awareness, about how research results are widely misinterpreted and over-simplified or without regard for the law-suits, problems with manufacturing, etc., drug advertising in the U.S. newspapers, magazines and on television continues to bring in loads of money for the profiteers. The problem has become so widespread that many health care and mental health professionals misunderstand the research as well. Many are not taught research design and analysis; many have no time to do the research and many only bother to read abstracts rather than understand the study. Still others simply rely on what the drug reps are taught to tell them. Apparently, health care in Europe, England and Canada is based on more accurate information, yet how many Canadians listen to the American ads?

See:
http://www.crisiscounseling.com/Articles/ExercisePositive%20Psychotherapy.htm

Antidepressants can help a few people. Journalists and advertisements incorrectly report that antidepressants can help up to 65% of people diagnosed with depression but when you read the research and account for placebo effects, you realize that 40 to 50% of depressed people would get better without an antidepressant. Only 15 to 25% improve somewhat on drugs. Research repeatedly confirms that 40 to 50% of depressed patients get better because of the passage of time, changes they make in their lives and fortunate events, and if you read all the studies on antidepressants you discover that nearly 6 out of 10 studies show that antidepressants don't work at all. The failed studies are never publicized and are often kept secret. In fact, the "new generation" of antidepressants (like Prozac) is not more effective than the previous generations of old ones. The new ones are just more expensive with different risks and side effects.

There are some important realities that are supported by research and publications.

- Many antidepressants require higher doses over time.

- Stopping antidepressants quickly, especially after years of use, can in some cases, be very unpleasant or even dangerous.

- Antidepressants, some more than others, can increase the risk of destructive, violent and suicidal behavior.

- The main differences among antidepressants are the side effects and allergic reactions.

- The more stimulating antidepressants, like Effexor, tend to be more addictive.

- Very few people will find one antidepressant more effective than another. (Some just make you feel worse than others.)

See:
http://www.crisiscounseling.com/Articles/ExercisePositive%20Psychotherapy.htm

Just a few weeks ago, an alarming report was released by the acclaimed New England Journal of Medicine proving once again that the pharmaceutical industry has entirely too much influence in Washington, D.C. and specifically with the Food and Drug Administration.

Bill Burniece of Panicyl wrote a beautiful but alarming article called: The Anti-depressant Scandal – Where is the Outrage? In the article he claimed that: "For the most part the antidepressant scandal has flown under the radar of most Americans. Perhaps most people missed the story with so much media attention focused on the heated presidential race."

His article explored how and why the "effectiveness of antidepressant drugs has been "severely over-hyped". The report reveals that pharmaceutical companies only publish the positive results and leave out the negative and/or fatal results. Apparently, when a drug company applies for a patent they only present the results that are in their favor and the physicians only hear about the positive results as well.

In reaction to various court cases that have revealed that anti-depressant studies showed a high incidence of suicidal ideation, suicidal behavior and completed suicides when on the anti-depressant resulting in the manufacturers being charged, (and other similar situations with other drugs) a law was passed in 2005 requiring complete disclosure of all results. While this sounds like a good remedy to a massive problem there is no one designated to monitor this abusive practice, so the practice continues. Furthermore, when negative analyses are actually presented, they are presented in such a manner that they actually appear to be positive in some way.

Many scientists are now realizing that if they write articles that denounce medications and show what the real research is saying, they will not get published. Thus, even if you have a good physician who is up to date on his journal reading, how is he going to have any more clarity than the physician who relies on what his pharmaceutical sales representative tells him or her?

As Bill Burniece claims, "This outrageous practice has major implications on our health. Since doctors rely primarily on this published medical journal data they are getting a skewed view of the effectiveness and safety of antidepressant drugs. As far as they know, little evidence exists to make them think twice about prescribing antidepressants to their patients. As a result, many more patients are ending up on frequently ineffective and dangerous antidepressant drugs."

So, why the outrage?

He questions our susceptibility and/or immunity to the greed and social irresponsibility that some of the major corporations have presented. Have we already forgotten the lessons taught by the likes of Enron, Tyco, Worldcom, and Adelphia?

Bill also questions the role of the FDA and other supposedly regulating bodies. They are funded by tax dollars but they are ruled by pharmaceutical companies, so who is really protecting the public?

Mr. Burniece further claims that Congress has

been well aware of the risks associated with antidepressants for many years. Yet, if they are aware, what have they done to address this huge issue? Just consider the political money that would be lost if Congress actually stood up and protected the people. Some claim that over 58% of the US Senate really represents pharmaceutical companies, not the people. Who controls the money? How much money? And at what cost?

Bill claims that the pharmaceutical industry consistently outspends other economic sectors on Washington lobbying. "Drug companies spent $155 million on lobbying between Jan 2005-June 2006. "What are the current numbers? What is the cost to your wallet? And more importantly what is the cost to your health?"

Bill claims that, "It's not just lobbying that keeps the pharmaceutical companies wealthy. Their bread and butter is consumer direct advertising. No surprise there. You can't turn on your television anymore without being bombarded by pharmaceutical ads plugging drugs for every ailment from osteoporosis to erectile dysfunction. No wonder more than half of all Americans are now on prescription medications."

See:
http://www.panicyl.com/Antidepressant_Sca
ndal.html

While I have referred to Bill Burniece's article
here as he presented a beautiful commentary,
there are loads of other articles, books, etc. that
claim the same issues. People just have to start
standing up and taking notice.

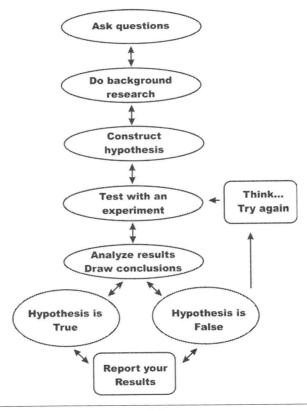

The challenge is that the ordinary person doesn't have training in research and design, statistical analysis, microbiology, amino acids, fatty acids, brain function/dysfunction, liver function/dysfunction, adrenal fatigue, gluta-thione, super oxide dismutase, and all the other steps required.

The average patient has no idea what he or she should be looking at, never mind having the time and the money required.

The only choice is simply to do what the doctor – who is probably almost as ignorant as they are of all the above – tells them to do which is what the pharmaceutical companies told the doctors to do.

We are going to now give you a summarized version of what different issues may be con-tributing to your depression or the depression in someone close to you. This will give you op-tions and choices and it will give you aware-ness.

This book is not meant to be either the assess-ment or treatment plan but rather designed to inform and make you aware of possible causes and options for treatment for depression.

THREE

So what are the causes of depression?

There are lots of known causes of depression. We will go through each one simply here in this chapter and then will elaborate on each in its own chapter.

The Psyche

We have a lot of research identifying how people interpret, respond to, and identify with the world and how that can cause major issues with depression.

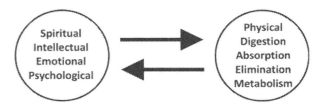

The psychological component of depression might be due to a lack of self-confidence or self-esteem; anger turned inwards or conflict in one's value systems. It might be due to underlying life themes that are working against you. It might be due to coping mechanisms or defense mechanisms that work against you rather than for you. These all might be age-old habits that you learned in childhood or somewhere along the way that simply became unconscious habits that you continue to engage in without realizing how detrimental they are.

Your Gut

Your gut is a fascinating component of your physical being. It actually exists outside of the body, i.e., it is a long tube within the body but go into the tube and you are outside of the body.

This fascinating tube actually has:

- its own nervous system
- contains between 90-95% of your entire immune system
- produces between 90-95% of the neuro-transmitter serotonin
- provides a breeding ground for over 800 different types of bacteria
- billions of bacteria.

The intestinal bacteria are not harmful but help with digestion and also play a protective role by forming a barrier around the intestine, thus preserving it from attacks by pathogenic organisms. However, if their development ceases to be regulated, they can proliferate and become pathogenic. The balance between these bacteria and the immune system controlling them is, therefore, essential.

See:
http://www.sciencedaily.com/releases/2008/11/081114185942.htm

If the gut leaks; or if it cannot break down nutrients; or if it cannot metabolize other nutrients; or if the bacteria get out of balance (either too many or too few); then any of these issues can impact on the rest of the body, including the brain, and can cause depression.

Hypothyroid

The hypothyroid syndrome or disorder is a very much confused and misunderstood issue. People, from the layperson to the psychologist to the family physician, are aware that hypothyroid involves TSH, T4, T3 and has an impact on energy, weight metabolism, and depression. However, how it works is vastly misunderstood.

Hypothyroid can actually involve the hypothalamus, the pituitary, the liver and the adrenals but who ever bothers to test any of these?

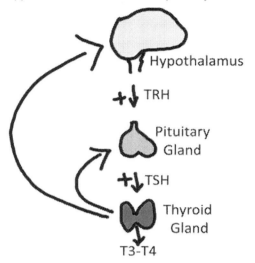

Hypothalamic - Pituitary - Thyroid Axis

Hypothalamus

+↓ TRH

Pituitary
Gland

+↓ TSH

Thyroid
Gland

T3-T4

TRH-Thyroid Releasing Hormone
TSH-Thyroid Stimulation Hormone

Adrenal Fatigue

The adrenals are little organs that sit on top of
the kidneys and produce a number of neurotransmitters and hormones and other molecules. These little organs jump into action
when we are stressed and overwhelmed...they
allow us the fight or flight response by shut-
ting down some systems and focusing all the
body energy into the necessary systems for
light or flight. If too overwhelmed, they will go
into the freeze response instead.

If the adrenals are either over-active or under-active they can cause a number of issues including depression.

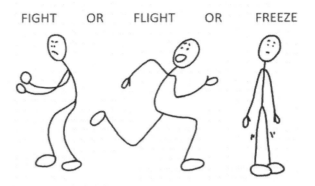

FIGHT   OR   FLIGHT   OR   FREEZE

Compromised Liver

Your liver is responsible for over 500 functions. Many of these functions support and protect the brain. If the liver doesn't function properly, this can cause depression.

Low Glutathione

Now you have probably heard about your adrenals and your thyroid before but have you ever heard of glutathione?
Let's first find out what glutathione does and then find out how to get more of it.

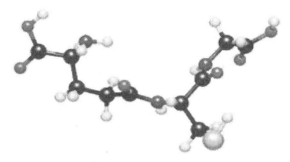

Glutathione Molecule

Master Anti-oxidant

Glutathione is considered the Master anti-oxidant for a variety of reasons:

- It is endogenous – made inside of the cell.

- It is a million times more powerful than any diet/supplementary anti-oxidant.

- It is the only anti-oxidant that re-stabilizes itself.

- It stabilizes all other anti-oxidants.

- Other anti-oxidants work on only one category of free radicals.

- Glutathione works on all groups of free radicals.

Other anti-oxidants work in one location.

Glutathione works in all locations:

- inside the cell
- in the cell membrane
- outside of the cell.

What are Free Radicals?

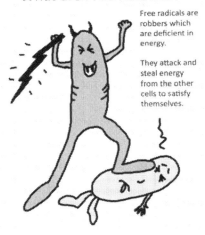

Free radicals are robbers which are deficient in energy.

They attack and steal energy from the other cells to satisfy themselves.

Detoxification

- Major component of Phase II in liver detoxification
- Major component of all cellular detoxification

Inflammation

- Major component of healthy inflammatory resolution

- With deficient levels inflammation becomes chronic and you develop fibrosis

Hormone regulation

- Involved either directly or indirectly with most hormones in the body

Cellular Energy

- Cells create ATP in the mitochondria for cellular energy
- Glutathione is the only known molecule that protects the mitochondria

Immune System

- Lymphocytes, i.e., T cells, B cells, macrophages, TNF, NK, etc. all require about 62% to both develop and function
- Regulates balance between different types of immune cells, for instance the balance between T1 and T2
- DNA, Cellular Transport
- Anti-aging, Calcium movement, respiratory

Regulates

- Nitric oxide = vasodilation
- Prostaglandin synthesis = vasodilation
- Hormones

DNA

- Protects the DNA from becoming cancerous
- Involved in both correction or elimination of abnormal DNA
- Required in protein synthesis

Cellular transport

- Required for most amino acid transportation in the cells

Anti-aging

- Like other anti-oxidants - prevents telomere breakdown
- Also the only known molecule that can provoke telomere creation
- Thus the only true anti-aging molecule

Calcium movement

- Required for regulation of Ca movement (required for muscle contraction in heart cells)

Respiratory

- 40% required in RBC to both pick up/release both O_2 & CO_2

Historically, we used to start making less glutathione around the age of 20. We lost about 1-2% per year and consequently were pretty low by the age of 90.

However, today we are losing between 12-15% per year and from the teen years on. Consequently by the age of 30 we are pretty depleted.

So let's look at the different issues that contribute to glutathione depletion:

- Age
- Drugs (alcohol, tobacco, legal and illegal drugs)
- Excess estrogens
- Exercising past a sweat
- Genetic abnormalities
- Household cleaners
- Infections
- Injuries

- Lack of hydration
- Metal toxicity
- Personal Hygiene products
- Pesticides, herbicides and certain food additives
- Pollution
- Poor diet
- Poor sleeping habits
- Radiation
- Stress
- Too much or too little sun

Glutathione has to be made inside of the cell – while you can take it as a food, a drink or a supplement, it will not increase your glutathione levels…but you will get expensive bowel movements. Considering most of us do not want to waste our money, we have to figure out how to get our bodies to make more glutathione inside the cells.

Glutathione is a tripeptide (3 proteins) and it breaks down into three amino acids in the gastro-intestinal tract (GIT). While we will absorb some of the amino acids, others are more likely to be lost with the bowels. Even if the glutathione stayed together as a whole molecule, there are no transport systems for glutathione into the cells.

What we need is all of the right nutrients

inside the cell so the cells can make glutathione. Unfortunately, some of these molecules are either in short supply in our food or difficult to get into the cells.

The most difficult of the three amino acids to get into the body and into the cell is the cysteine. It is a very difficult molecule to keep stable and has to be connected to a thiol and a hydrol. About 15 years ago, a scientist patented a way to stabilize cysteine to help the cellular production of glutathione and in fact showed an increase of glutathione production about 15-30%.

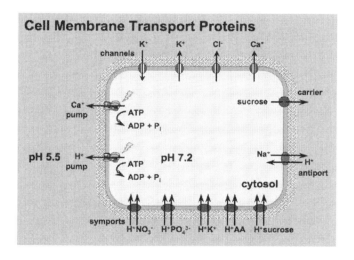

Today, however, there is a patented composition that has shown an average increase of 292% in two months for the average person. What makes this a particularly unique product is that it is like a pancake mix. It has all the necessary ingredients, in the right ratios, to make glutathione effectively within the cell. (It is called OGF – Original Glutathione Formula. See: www.choicesunlimited.ca/OGF.)

In addition, we now have a five-herb formulation that turns on the genetic tools to make glutathione, i.e., mRNA. Science has now identified between 5,000 and 6,000 genes of our 25,000 genes that are considered the "survival mechanisms" of every cell.

This herb formulation turns on the anti-inflammatory pathways, the anti-fibrosis pathways and the anti-oxidant pathways, of these survival mechanisms, consisting of: Glutathione (increase of 300% within one month).

- Super Oxide Dismutase (SOD) (68% increase).

- Catalase (25% increase).

- Turning the cell's survival mechanisms back on again allows the body to function at its optimal level – in all systems.

This increase in glutathione addresses all the toxins, metals, inflammatory, fibrotic, issues in the body and increases the body's functioning in the following systems:

- Central nervous systems
- Respiratory systems
- Immune systems
- Cardiovascular systems
- Liver system
- Kidney system

All these systems can have an impact on the brain and the brain's capacity to function effectively. If the brain is not functioning effectively, depression can be the result.

FOUR

The Psychology of Depression

We know from psychology that depression can be caused from how we interpret and respond to the world, however, after practicing as a registered psychologist for 20 years I was convinced that most females who suffered "depression" were really suffering from "frustration".

Why would I say that? For example, women get frustrated when their partners act like children rather than adults. When women are contributing significantly to the household finances but their partners are not contributing significantly to:

- parenting the children
- looking after the ailing parents
- taking care of the laundry, cooking, cleaning, vacuuming, dusting, etc.

When a woman's partner gets to spend time and money playing golf because they "need time to themselves" but never think their wives need to take time for themselves, that's frustrating.

When they are stuck in abusive relationships and cannot see how they can get out or stuck in jobs they hate and cannot find a way out women become enormously frustrated but often have no outlet for their feelings. When they feel disrespected, undervalued, or insignificant in their homes or jobs or when their partners are alcoholics, drug addicts, gamblers, sex and/or affair addicts, etc. what is a woman to do?

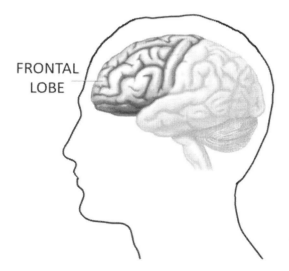

FRONTAL
LOBE

Now, that is not to say that external situations are always the cause. A woman may be causing her own frustration out of:

- Fear of leaving a bad situation.

- The belief that "the devil they know is better than the devil they don't know".

- Fear that they couldn't put food on the table or a roof over the heads of their children if they left, etc.

On the other hand, frustration may also be the result of not effectively interpreting and responding to the world. For instance, a person may engage in various thought patterns, some of which are known as Beck's Cognitive Distortions, which include:

- Minimizing or maximizing inappropriately, i.e., "making a mountain out of a molehill" or "catastrophizing" or focusing on just the negative or just the positive.

- All or none thinking, i.e., utilizing concepts like always, every, never, etc. rather than recognizing that it is probably sometimes, occasionally, perhaps, or maybe.

- Overgeneralization, i.e. taking one example and applying it without discernment to all situations.

- Mental filtering, i.e. inability to see the bigger picture or the whole process. For instance, noticing only the small imperfection on a piece of clothing as opposed to the whole piece.

- Jumping to conclusions, i.e. reaching a conclusion on one piece of evidence rather than looking at all sides.

- Mind reading – perception that you understand the intentions of others when in fact you are simply projecting your thoughts, attitudes, etc. onto them.

- Fortune-telling – inflexible expectations for how things will turn out before they happen.

- Emotional reasoning, i.e. "I feel it, therefore it must be real", drawing conclusions, making decisions, etc. based on what you feel rather than on actual data.

- Rigid thinking, i.e. thinking in terms of "should" or "ought to" or living by a set of rules that you apply regardless of the situation, rather than dealing with each specific situation with objectivity.

- Labeling/mislabeling, i.e. limited thinking about behaviors or events due to a reliance on names or labels – tends to be highly colored and emotionally loaded.

- Personalization – taking responsibility for people, situations, etc. over which you have no control.

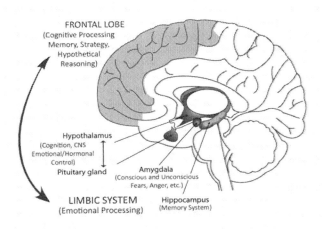

As you can see there are lots of psychological layers that may have an impact on the experience of depression.

Now let's look at some of the other issues.

FIVE

Understanding your gut and its relationship to depression

It has been well established in alternative medicines and throughout history in various cultural healing beliefs that the gut has an impact far beyond digestion. It is only now being recognized in the Western science.

Unfortunately, Western research always seems to be far behind what alternative healing has known for seemingly thousands of years. However, it is now recognized that gut health is directly related to bone formation, liver health, cardiovascular systems, allergies and all kinds of brain issues, such as learning, memory, Parkinson's disease, depression, and more.

Recent research has recognized that disruptions to both the stomach health and intestinal bacteria can promote depression and anxiety in lab creatures. Just like anxiety, a cognitive or mental issue can cause an upset stomach.

"The gut is important in medical research, not just for problems pertaining to the digestive system but also problems pertaining to the rest of the body," says Pankaj J. Pasricha, Chief of the Division of Gastroenterology and Hepatology at Stanford University School of Medicine.

So, let's look at this concept that the gut is considered the second brain. Physiologically, the gut — which stems from the esophagus, through the stomach, the small and large intestines to the rectum — has its own nervous system that allows it to operate independently from the brain. Like the brain and spinal cord, the gut is filled with nerve cells.

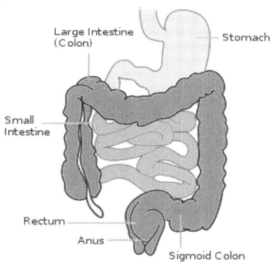

The small intestine alone has 100 million neurons, roughly equal to the amount found in the spinal cord, says Dr. Michael Gershon, professor of pathology and cell biology at Columbia University.

See:
http://gut.bmj.com/content/39/4/551.abstract

This digestive system is also called the enteric nervous system and is referred to as the "gut brain". It can operate independently of the brain. It produces neurotransmitters also found in the brain, for instance, and produces 90-95% of the serotonin found in the body.

The vagus nerve is the tenth cranial nerve out of twelve and stretches down from the brain stem through the trunk of the body. The vagus nerve is the main connection between the brain and gut but the gut doesn't just take orders from the brain.

"The brain is a CEO that doesn't like to micromanage," says Dr. Gershon. The brain receives much more information from the gut than it sends down, he adds.

Another research study found that electrically stimulating the Vagus nerve – which controls the gut – reduced the symptoms of epilepsy and depression. (One treatment approved by the U.S. Food and Drug Administration, made by Cyberonics Inc. is already on the market.)

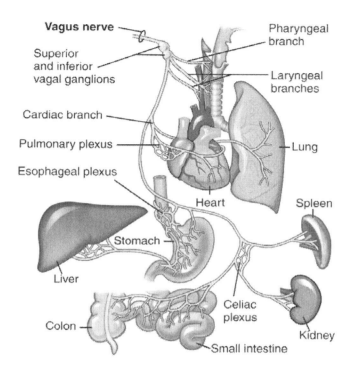

Vagus nerve

Pharyngeal branch

Superior and inferior vagal ganglions

Laryngeal branches

Cardiac branch

Pulmonary plexus

Lung

Esophageal plexus

Heart

Spleen

Stomach

Liver

Colon

Celiac plexus

Kidney

Small intestine

Similarly, it has been found that this kind of stimulation helps improve learning and memory.

We have long known that the digestive tract controls organs including the pancreas and gall bladder via nerve connections. We have also long known that hormones and neurotransmitters generated and secreted in the gut interact with organs such as the lungs and heart and bones and the liver.

But the gut can also have a direct impact on the brain.

Many people with psychiatric and brain conditions report also having gastrointestinal issues. Research indicates that problems in the GI Tract may cause problems in the brain, just as a mental ailment, such as anxiety, can upset the stomach. There is a lot of research showing that patients with depression and anxiety also often have bowel symptoms, i.e. irritable bowel syndrome.

Dr. Pasricha and colleagues, of Stanford University, explored the brain-gut connection in the lab by irritating the stomachs of newborn rats. They found that by the age of ten weeks, while the physical irritation issue had been resolved, they displayed more depressed and anxious behaviors, such as giving up more quickly in a swimming task, than rats whose stomachs weren't irritated.

Compared to controls, the rats also showed increased sensitivity to stress and produced more of a stress hormone, in a study published in May in a Public Library of Science Journal, PLoS One.

The conclusions of another research study with humans claimed:

"These objective measurements of intestinal transit in affective disorders (mood disorders) are consistent with clinical impressions that anxiety is associated with increased bowel frequency, and depressed patients tend to be constipated; mood has an effect on intestinal motor function."

Source:
http://gut.bmj.com/content/39/4/551.abstract

Now it gets even more interesting. In the human body there are 10 to the 12th number of cells, give or take, but there are an estimated 10 to the 13th number of cells that are not us, i.e. bacteria, fungus, yeast, etc. In particular, in the small intestine, there are over 350 different species of bacteria that we require and there are over 475 known species in the large intestine.

Another study of 23 autistic children and 9 typically developing kids found that those with autism had a unique bacterium called Sutterella.

Now we go to researchers from McMaster University in Hamilton, Ontario, who demonstrated that bacteria in the gut, a.k.a. gut flora, play a role in how the body responds to stress. While the exact mechanism is unknown, certain bacteria are thought to facilitate important interactions between the gut and the brain.

Dr. Gershon, professor of pathology and cell biology at Columbia University has been studying how the gut controls its behavior and that of other organs by investigating the neurotransmitter serotonin.

Low serotonin levels in the brain have long been thought to affect mood and sleep, although this has not been proven. Yet, several common antidepressants work, supposedly, by raising levels of serotonin in the brain.

On the other hand, serotonin and other neurotransmitters produced by gut neurons help the digestive tract to metabolize and/or move food through the gut. Serotonin seems to play a role in motility, sensitivity and secretion of fluids and the amount of fluid in stools.

Could it be that when people are given antidepressants, at least when they appear to work, it is actually because of the activity in the gut as opposed to the brain?

Source:
http://online.wsj.com/article/SB10001424052
97020446800457716473294974356.html

SIX

Misconceptions of Hypothyroid and Depression

As mentioned above, the hypothyroid syndrome or disorder is a very much confusing and misunderstood issue. Hypothyroid can actually involve the hypothalamus, the pituitary, the liver and the adrenals. But who ever bothers to test any of these? Further, T3 and T4 can have a huge impact on the brain.

Let's start with the thyroid. The thyroid is one of the largest endocrine (hormone) glands and is situated in the neck. The thyroid is now recognized as having a much more important role in the health of your metabolic endocrine, nervous and immune systems.

These systems in turn have an important role in the health and optimal functioning of your brain, including cognitive functions, such as the ability to concentrate, memory and attention span, and emotion/mood stability.

However, there is a huge misconception about the thyroid and the hypothyroid condition which is often thought to cause depressive symptoms, particularly in women.

THE THYROID FEEDBACK LOOP

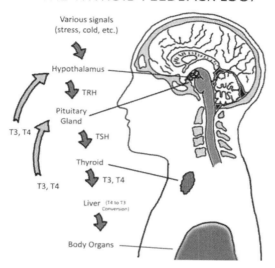

The process of stimulating the thyroid begins in the hypothalamus in the brain, which releases TRH (thyroid releasing hormone) which sends a message to the pituitary to release TSH (thyroid stimulating hormone). TSH stimulates the thyroid to produce T4 and T3 in the follicular cells.

Now, what happens in the thyroid? While most epithelial cells are usually non-vascularized cells (meaning no blood nutrient support), the epithelial cells in the thyroid form clusters that function as glands which are usually vascularized (they take up nutrients from the blood and release the subsequent hormones into the blood flow).

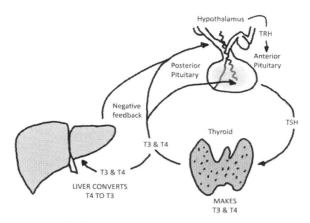

The epithelial cells of the thyroid take up iodine and amino acids from the blood and make thyroglobulin and thyro-peroxidase. These nutrients are released into the thyroid follicles along with iodine. Then with the help of proteases, the thyroid follicles make T4 (80%) and T3 (20%).

The T3 is about four times more powerful than the T4, so we want more of it. However, we can transform T4 into T3 and about 80% of that conversion happens in the liver, not the thyroid. This conversion requires iodinases, an enzyme.

To complicate things, however, these iodinases

can be blocked from action by cortisol secreted from the adrenals. But let's go back to T3 and T4 for a moment.

THYROID SYSTEM

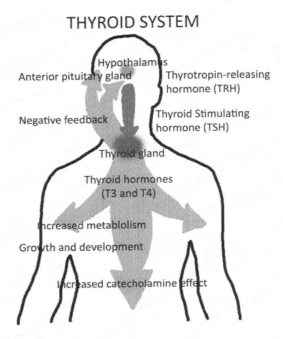

T3 and T4 are circulated by the blood (by attaching to globulins – transporters) to every cell in the body. These hormones connect to cell receptors, whereby they gain access to the cells.

These hormones regulate the rate of metabolism (conversion of oxygen and calories to energy) and affect the rate of growth and rate of function in cells and therefore, in many systems in the body.

Every cell in the body actually depends upon thyroid hormones for these metabolic functions.

What becomes really important here is that brain cells have more T3 receptors than any other tissue!

See:
http://www.stopthethyroidmadness.com/thyroid-depression-mental-health/

Historically, it was believed that only T4 crossed the blood-brain barrier (BBB) but Dr. John Lowe claims that this is an old false belief that people simply won't let go of.

"Transthyretin" is the protein that transports T4 across the blood-brain barrier. It also transports T3 across. It may transport less T3, however, because the binding affinity of the receptors within the protein is about ten times less for T3 than for T4."

Dr. Lowe claims that unfortunately, "Transthyretin also transports chemical contaminants such as dioxins and PCBs across the (blood-brain) barrier." As we know, these are not good chemicals to have, in general, but specifically here, the problem is that these toxic chemicals displace T4 and T3 from the thyroid hormone receptors inside the transthyretin molecule, meaning that our hormones don't trigger the cells.

Now we have to remember that virtually all humans are polluted with contaminants. Toxicologists claim that we have all these particular contaminants - T4 and T3 displacement may be a major mechanism of health problems from a brain deficiency of thyroid hormone.

Dr. Lowe continues: "The potential health problems from this displacement are highly complex... after contaminants displace T4 and T3 from transthyretin, bind to the hormone receptors in the protein, and then ride the protein into the brain, the contaminants can bind to thyroid hormone receptors on genes. The binding alters the normal transcription activities of the genes, producing adverse effects that are hard to predict and diagnose."

So to sum up:

- the belief that T3 doesn't cross the blood-brain barrier is false.
- the documentation is far from new.
- we need to address this and help physicians and patients understand what is really going on.

See:
http://www.drlowe.com/jcl/comentry/t3entersbrain.htm

http://www.thyroidscience.com/

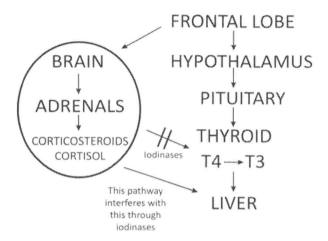

Okay, so now that we know T3 and T4 get into the brain, what exactly do they do? Well, T3 is very important to the brain for:

1. Maturation

2. Influences neural cell migration (movement to specific areas)

3. Cell differentiation (all cells start from stem cells, but each needs to develop into a unique kind of cell)

4. Signaling (communication between cells)

5. The expression of genes in myelination (the myelination is the insulation of the trunk of a neuron – if it gets depleted, you suffer multiple sclerosis). Genes (DNA) may remain the same throughout life but they are off/on switches. Many molecules in our bodies and in our food, can affect whether given switches are OFF or ON.

See: http://www.ncbi.nlm.nih.gov/pubmed/16112266

Further, T3 acts as hormone in the following kinds of cells:

- Glial cells (the maintenance crew of the brain).

- Astrocytes (play a role in structural, metabolic, neurotransmitter release, blood flow and repair work).

- Tanyctes (special cells that extend into the hypothalamus and link to neural hormones and enzymes).

- Oligodendrocytes (like Schwann cells they provide insulation to neural axons [the trunk of the neuron] but whereas Schwann cells provide insulation to only one neuron; olgiodendrocytes can provide insulation to 50 different axons at the same time).

Let's sum up what we have said so far.

The hypothalamus sends a hormone to the pituitary.

The pituitary sends a hormone to the thyroid. The thyroid then makes predominantly T4.

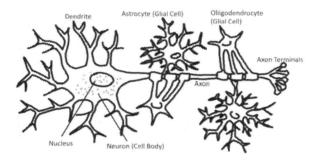

The liver does most of the conversion of T4 to T3 conversion which is much more powerful – but if the adrenals are producing cortisol then that interferes with the liver conversion.

We also know that T3 plays a number of different roles in a wide variety of cells in the brain. So, if we don't have enough T3, we can suffer depression.

We are not sure why we are still calling this hypothyroid – but hey, why not? What we do know is that like most things that happen in the body it requires an entire system and the system is interactive with other systems.

Another component is that usually, the system has gone through "hyperthyroid" functioning before it ends up in a "hypothyroid" functioning process.

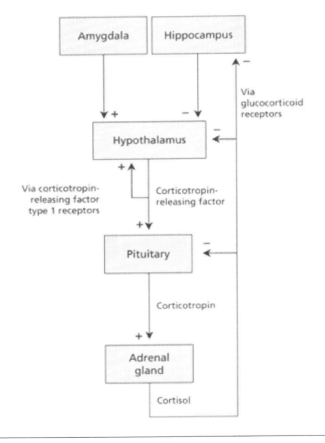

Synthroid

Now let's take a brief look at the drug called Synthroid. This drug is a synthetic replacement for a lack of T4. It is not an active hormone. So, what happens when your doctor diagnoses you as hypothyroid is, first of all, rather than address your compromised adrenals and liver, he or she is just going to give you an artificial medication hoping that the body will convert the T4 to T3.

The challenge is that while Synthroid may help some people in the short term, .i.e., while their body is recovering from stress, in the long run it apparently does something else.

Under normal conditions your body produces a small amount of rT3 which binds to the T3 cell receptors and prevents absorption of T3 into the cell. This isn't a problem unless the body is in a stress response – which is usually what caused the "hypothyroid" issue in the first place.

Under the stress response, the cortisol prevents the iodinases from converting T4 to T3 in the liver. Consequently, there is even less conversion of T4 to T3 in the liver. Furthermore, cortisol enhances the conversion of the T4 to rT3. So now not only do we have the cortisol working against us, but we also have the rT3 working against us. This is called rT3 dominance.

In addition, there is a feedback loop that causes even more of an issue. The Synthroid T4 provokes an excess which tells the pituitary not to produce TSH - this stops the production of T4 and T3 in the thyroid. And now, with the higher levels of T4 (which is actually just Synthroid) the body converts the T4 to rT3, which blocks the T3 receptors even further. This ends up causing even more of the original "hypothyroid" issues than you started with.

Other issues that are also known to cause rT3 dominance are:

- Fasting (including repeated weight loss diets)
- Surgery
- Burn trauma
- Alcoholism
- Endotoxin injections
- Clinical glucocorticoids (cortisone shots and prednisone therapy)

So if we go back to the brain function, we have more rT3 and less T3. This affects the metabolic function of all the different types of maintenance crews in the brain that are required for effective neural functioning. Do you not think this might cause a sense of depression – with a wide variety of different expressions?

SEVEN

Adrenal Fatigue and Depression

The adrenals are two glands that sit on top of your kidneys. The right one is more of a triangular shaped organ and the left is more of a semi-lunar shape. The inside component is called the medulla and the outer component is the cortex. Each part synthesizes (produces) and secretes (releases) hormones.

The adrenals are well known for their response to the flight-fight stress response – this is when the cortex releases corticosteroids such as cortisol, and hormones, and the medulla releases catecholamines such as epinephrine and norepinephrine, which are neurotransmitters.

Right Adrenal Gland   Left Adrenal Gland

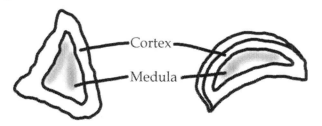

The adrenal cortex has three layers each of which produces its own hormones:

- The outside layer produces mineral-corticoids like aldosterone (blood pressure).

- The middle layer produces the glucocorticoids like cortisol (flight-fight response).

- The inside layer produces androgens like DHEA (required for both testosterone and the estrogens) and a host of other functions the understanding of which is still controversial.

The adrenal medulla secretes about 20% norephinephrine and 80% epinephrine, both of which are neurotransmitters. The medulla receives direction through the sympathetic nervous system (the activating component of the central nervous system directed from the brain).

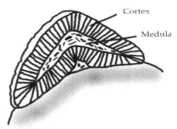

What does any of this have to do with mood disorders? Well, quite a lot actually. When one is under stress and produces these corticosteroids they are difficult to get rid of and it takes a lot of time. In our stressful society, we tend to live on these corticosteroids just to keep going at our hectic pace. The body can't get rid of them and they turn into free radicals which end up causing destruction of healthy molecules and cells. The body desperately struggles to get rid of these harmful free radicals by using up the anti-oxidants.

This not only depletes our body's natural anti-oxidants but also the anti-oxidants we take in through our diet and supplements. (Note the body's master anti-oxidant, glutathione, is a million times more powerful than any anti-oxidant you might find in your diet or supplements. It also appears that glutathione is involved in more functions in your body than almost any other molecule.)

So with the increase of free radicals, we deplete glutathione. With the depletion of glutathione, the liver does not function effectively.

When the liver does not function effectively it cannot support the brain. So now, we are having a challenge with the adrenals, the liver the gut (don't forget the liver helps supports the gut which we are already recognized had a big impact on the brain) and the brain.

What is important to note is that after a period of time adrenal fatigue sets in (although in some situations it may set in very fast) and one needs to be careful.

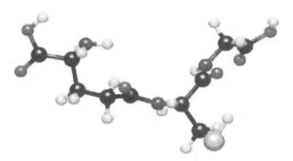

Glutathione Molecule

The following symptoms are associated with adrenal fatigue syndrome:

- Cravings for salty, fatty, high protein foods, i.e. meat, cheese and nuts.
- Decreased memory capacity.
- Difficulties getting up in the morning.
- Feeling better suddenly for a brief period after a meal.
- Feeling better when stress is relieved, such as during vacations.
- High frequency of getting the flu and/ or other respiratory diseases.

- Increased PMS symptoms – periods heavy with sudden stops and starts.

- Lack of energy in the morning and between 3:00 and 5:00 p.m.

- Lightheaded when rising from a horizontal position.

- Often tired between 9:00 and 10:00 p.m. but resist going to bed.

- Pain in the upper back and/or neck with no explanation.

- Reduced sexual drive.

- Tendency to gain weight and inability to lose it, especially around the waist.

- Use coffee or stimulants to get going in the morning.

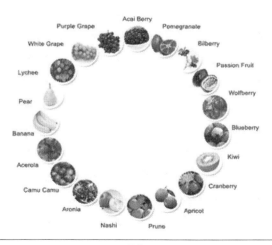

In addition, other symptoms might include:

- Alternating constipation and diarrhea.
- Decreased ability to handle stress.
- Dry and thin skin.
- Dyspepsia or indigestion.
- Food and/or inhalant allergies.
- Hypoglycemia.
- Increased effort to perform daily tasks.
- Lethargy and lack of energy.
- Low body temperature.
- Mild depression.
- Nervousness.
- Heart palpitations.
- Unexplained hair loss.

We said previously that the adrenals and thyroid work in concert and one should not be treated without the other so now let's do a brief summary of why this is the case.

Remember, the hypothalamus releases TRH which stimulates the pituitary to release TSH which provokes the thyroid to make 80%T4 and 20% T3. 80% of the T4 -> T3 conversion happens in the liver; and T3 is four times more powerful than T4 but if one is stressed, especially for a period of time, the cortisol that the adrenals secretes block the T4 – T3 conversion and allows more rT3 to be made thereby blocking the receptors on cells.

Now cellular metabolism doesn't happen; conversion of calories and oxygen into energy doesn't happen and a whole long list of other things do not happen.

We need to help strengthen both the adrenals and the thyroid – and actually, the liver, too, but we will address the liver in Chapter Eight on Detoxification.

References:

http://www.royalrife.com/0103.html
http://en.wikipedia.org/wiki/RT3
http://www.wilsonssyndrome.com/armour-or-synthroid/

EIGHT

Compromised Liver and Depression

The skin is considered the largest organ of the body and certainly has the largest surface area of all organs (weighs in at about 15% of the total body weight) and certainly performs a lot of functions.

The liver, however, is the largest internal organ and is definitely larger in terms of weight and number of functions. Its complexity is only second to the brain.

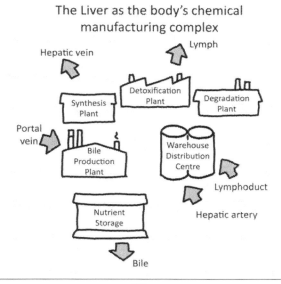

The Liver as the body's chemical manufacturing complex

These functions help to support every other organ and system in the body so if the gut has an impact on the liver the impact is huge.

The liver is largest organ (3.2-3.7 lbs. or 1.4-1.7 kg) inside the body and carries out over 500 functions including:

1. Vascular (blood management).

2. Provides blood clotting factors.

3. Filters the blood and helps remove harmful chemicals and bacteria with glutathione to detoxify.

4. Stores extra blood to be quickly released when needed.

5. Removes damaged and old red blood cells.

6. Helps to maintain blood pressure.

7. Constructs cholesterol, testosterone, estrogen, and reconstructs hormones.

8. Produces coagulation factors, bile, insulin-like growth factor thrombopoietin (necessary for the productions of platelets in bone marrow).

9. Metabolizes proteins, fats, and carbohydrates thus providing energy and nutrients.

10. Helps to assimilate and store fat soluble vitamins (A, E, D, and K).

11. Stores vitamins, minerals, and sugars.

12. Creates bile which gets stored in the gall bladder and which breaks down fats in the gut.

13. Creates blood serum proteins which maintain fluid balance and act as carriers (transporters).

14. Helps maintain electrolytes and water balance.

15. Creates immune substances such as gamma globulin.

16. Breaks down and eliminates excess hormones, such as insulin.

17. Breaks down ammonia (and other toxins) created in the colon by bacteria thus preventing death.

18. Humanizes nutrients, metabolizes protein, carbohydrates, fat for energy.

19. Synthesizes urea, constructs blood protein, interconverts amino acids.

20. Constructs 50,000 systems of enzymes to govern metabolic activity throughout the body.

21. Metabolizes drugs.

See:
http://en.wikipedia.org/wiki/Liver

http://www.pacifichealth.com/protocols/live
r.html

http://en.wikipedia.org/wiki/Red_blood_cell
s
http://www.livestrong.com/article/17243-
depression-caused-liver-disease/

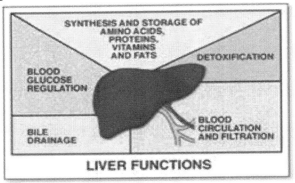

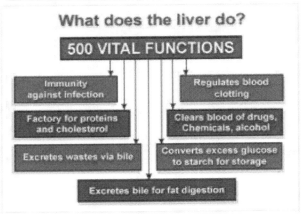

A problem with any one of these processes can cause problems with the brain.

1. Glutathione is an extremely important molecule in every cell of the body perhaps with more functions than any other molecule in the body. Certainly, it is involved in almost every system, whether directly or indirectly. This molecule is called the Master Anti-oxidant. The reason for this is predominantly because of two reasons:

a) it can address all categories of free radicals.

b) it recycles itself and all other types of anti-oxidants.

Consider these facts about glutathione.

- It is involved in most of the body's detox pathways at both a cellular level and in the liver.

- It detoxifies the blood and/or prepares molecules to be eliminated through the kidneys.

- It is the body's primary chelator, i.e. drawing toxic metals from the blood.

- It is involved with the anti-inflammatory pathways.

- It is required for the immune system to both develop and to respond.

- It is also required for the respiratory system to take up and release both oxygen and carbon dioxide.

- It regulates NO (nitric oxide) an important messaging molecule that is involved extensively in vasodilation, the immune system and the neurological system.

- It regulates a wide number of hormones directly or indirectly through NO.

If glutathione levels are low, the liver gets sluggish and heavy, which results in poor circulation and poor oxygen delivery, to all parts of the body and in particular to the brain. This sluggishness results in cells, tissues, and the brain becoming undernourished, an increase of oxidative stress and a resulting inflammatory process.

When the brain becomes overloaded with toxins, an increase in oxidative stress occurs and a resulting increase in inflammation occurs. When this happens, the brain cannot function effectively which causes all kinds of issues from depression to bipolar to schizophrenia.

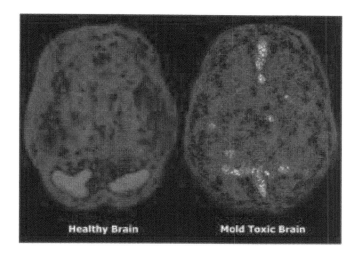

Healthy Brain   Mold Toxic Brain

2. The liver plays an important role in the rejuvenation of red blood cells. This is a very important for the entire body because if the liver cannot rejuvenate red blood cells effectively then oxygen cannot get to the rest of the body and to the brain. While this function is important to all parts of the body, it is particularly important to the brain because the various different types of glial cells in the brain rely on oxygen to function and transport oxygen to the neurons. Glial cells (the brain maintenance crew) also:

- surround neurons and hold them in place

- insulate the neurons from one another

- destroy pathogens in the brain and re-move dead neurons

- participate in the movement of neuro-transmitters

- release important molecules like ATP (the fuel for most functions in every cell).

Thus, if the liver cannot make sure that oxygen gets to the brain, a lot of functions are going to go amiss in the brain causing issues like depression.

3. With an excess of copper in the liver, one develops Wilson's disease which affects the central nervous system and can result in neu-rological symptoms like depression.

Liver disease is not actually just one disease but rather a collection of diseases, infections and conditions that affect the ability of the liver cells to function.

The stages of alcohol-induced liver damage:

Fatty Liver
- Deposits of fat causes liver enlargement.
- Strict abstinence can lead to a full recov-ery.

Liver Fibrosis
- Scar tissue forms.
- Recovery is possible, but scar tissue remains.

Cirrhosis
- Growth of connective tissue destroys liver cells.
- The damage is irreversible.

Research regarding liver disease is very alarming. Statistics suggest that by the time one is 30 years old, the liver is functioning at 75% of capacity. Liver toxicity and inflammation results in injury then fibrosis and finally, cirrhosis.

There are apparently over a 100 recognized forms of liver disease that may lead to cirrhosis of the liver. NAFLD (non-alcoholic fatty liver disease which is histologically indistinguishable from alcoholic liver diseases) is now being seen regularly in children. This correlates with the increase in obesity and diabetes in children.

Liver Function Tests

GGT/(5GGT)	Increased with alcoholic Hepatitis or biliary stasis	Increased with alcoholic cirrhosis or biliary cirrhosis
Total Bilirubin	Normal if the Hepatitis is due to other causes	Normal if the cirrhosis is due to other causes
Bilirubin-D	Normal or increased	Normal or increased
Bilirubin-1	Bilirubin-D is > bilirubin-I in most cases	Bilirubin-I is > bilirubin-D in most cases

Source:
http://books.google.ca/books?id=SB_-
CRXvZPYC&pg=PA1241&dq=NAFLD+statisti
cs&hl=en&sa=X&ei=MW53T5ifPIvKiQLF58mn
Dg&ved=0CFUQ6AEwBg#v=onepage&q

There's an old saying in China that goes, "If you're depressed, blame the liver." Chinese medicine believes there is a direct correlation between liver function and depression. Their findings are based, at least in part, in fact.

The Chinese have found that drugs such as tranquilizers, sleeping pills and antihistamines weaken the liver. This weakening of the liver results in what they call liver depression, a condition which actually refers to your liver's ability to function as opposed to your psychological state of mind. However, if the liver's functioning is depressed it can result in your brain's inability to function which may mean depression for you.

Read more:
http://www.livestrong.com/article/17243-
depression-caused-liver-
disease/#ixzz1qZPCZK00

Liver disease impedes the body's ability to process Vitamin B compounds. The consequence of making low levels of vitamin Bs is the inability to make SAMe (S-

Adenosylmethionine) which is a key molecule that prevents depression.

As you can see, a compromised liver has an enormous capacity to create an experience of depression.

References:
http://www.livestrong.com/article/17243-depression-caused-liver-disease/
http://healthmad.com/conditions-and-diseases/sluggish-liver-creates-depression/

NINE

Deficient levels of Glutathione and Depression

We have looked at some of the important organs that have an impact on depression. Now we are going to explore some nutrients and their impact on depression.

We have already explored some aspects of glutathione in terms of liver functioning. Now let's look at glutathione, or the lack thereof, on the brain's functioning.

Glutathione is the most abundant protein-like substance in the brain. It helps prevent impaired functions and death of nerve cells in a variety of ways by eliminating excess NMDA (a neuroexcitatory and inflammatory creating substance).

See:
http://www.chemicalinjury.net/html/neural_sensitization-pg_6.html

The cells in the human brain consume approximately 20% of the oxygen utilized by the body despite the fact that it makes up for about 2%

of the body's weight. Thus, the rate of reactive oxygen species, or ROS, or free radicals is very high in the brain.

As noted previously, glutathione is the Master Anti-oxidant. This master anti-oxidant is then hugely important for the brain as well. We know that the highest levels of glutathione are found in the liver, probably due to its necessity in the detoxifying processes but now we find that the second highest levels are in the brain, again, perhaps because of the need for detoxification processes.

The glutathione detoxification system involves two types of glutathione called the (GSSG/GSH) redox system. Glutathione essentially separates into two molecules; it gives away electrons and then with the help of enzymes, comes back together again, so that it can do the process all over again with another free radical. Note this is a very simplistic story as the glutathione complex is actually made up of various different components, for example, 8 different glutathione peroxidases but you don't need to know all that.)

We know glutathione is involved in a huge number of processes in the body but now we also know that it does a wide variety of specialized functions in the brain. For instance, it regulates the activity of a variety of different proteins through different enzyme processes, i.e. Glutathionylation. (Thank goodness, you don't need to know what that means!) The long and short of it is that through different pathways (protein phosphatases, protein kinases and transcription factors) glutathione has a huge impact on neural functioning.

See:
http://www.ncbi.nlm.nih.gov/pubmed/17034341

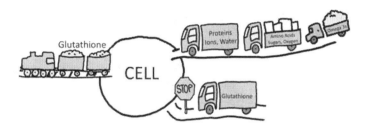

Nitric Oxide is an important molecule, actually a gas, which is involved in vasodilation, the expansion of arteries. Glutathione regulates Nitric Oxide (NO), so glutathione is important in the brain, as it is throughout the entire body, to allow for expansion in the arteries. If the arteries do not expand, the blood flow does not reach the cells; the cells do not get nourishment, and of course, we have hypertension. With lack of proper blood flow, toxins are also not removed.

One theory on neural function suggests that glutathione accumulates during the day during "waking metabolism" and induces sleep by enhancing GABA (the primary inhibitory neurotransmitter in the brain and required for sleep processes).

See:
http://alturl.com/899c7

Glutathione is also thought to be a neurohormone in the brain which means it sends signals from one part of the brain to another. In addition, glutathione stimulates and regulates different types of glial cells (astrocytes). It is also believed that glutathione might be involved in the function of various hormones in the brain.

Also see:
http://www.scribd.com/doc/2325470/Metabolism-and-Functions-of-Glutathione-in-Brain

http://www.chemicalinjury.net/html/neural_sensitization-pg_6.html

One can easily see that a molecule with such important and diverse roles would have a huge impact on the brain if there was a deficiency. One of these impacts has been shown to be both cognitive and mood disorders.

TEN

Deficient Levels of Magnesium and Depression

Magnesium is a mineral that plays a major role in the body. Magnesium plays a repeated role in the required cell processes to make the fuel for the cells, called ATP (adenosine triphosphate).

This alone makes magnesium important. The fuel is required for virtually all enzyme processes, i.e. to break anything down or build anything up we need enzymes and fuel.

Consequently, magnesium is required for over 300 known enzyme functions in every cell in the body, never mind a wide variety of specialty processes. For instance, it is required to connect cartilage synovial mesenchymal stem cells. Synovial mesenchymal cells are special cells that differentiate into connective tissue, i.e., bone, cartilage, tendon, etc. Once developed, these cells need to adhere to cartilage to repair damage and magnesium is required to facilitate this process.

Magnesium is the fourth most abundant element in the brain and is required for a variety of functions in the brain:

- It protects the brain from toxic effects of chemicals such as food additives.
- It is a natural blood thinner, preventing clots, strokes, blood vessel spasms and pain.
- It relaxes the head and neck muscle tension (required for relaxation in all muscles) that make migraines worse.
- It is involved in brain metabolism.
- It regulates central nervous system excitability.

Symptoms of low neural magnesium include:

- Anorexia
- Anxiety
- Apathy
- Apprehension
- Confusion
- Depression
- Dizziness
- Epilepsy type convulsions
- Fatigue
- Insomnia
- Irritability
- Loss of appetite

- Muscle tremors
- Nervousness
- Poor memory
- Twitching

See:
http://members.upnaway.com/~poliowa/Ma
gnesium%20-%20a%20Miracle.html
http://www.fi.edu/learn/brain/micro.html

There are twelve different types of magnesium. Only three are bioavailable though there remain various controversies over which are the most bioavailable. It is important to consult a health care practitioner to determine which is best for a given situation.

In conclusion, one can understand why a lack of magnesium might cause various expressions of depression.

ELEVEN

Deficiency in B Vitamins and Depression

The B Vitamins are involved in making energy, just like magnesium is, and are also involved in neural functioning. In fact, typically where B1, B2, and/or B3 are utilized in the pathways to make ATP, you also find magnesium.

Vitamin B1 or Thiamine is also essential for a variety of other biochemical reactions. For instance, B1 is involved in the:

- synthesis of neuro-enzymes (deficiency prevents metabolism of glucose for fuel)

- neurotransmitters – serotonin, norephinephrine, dopamine, acetylcholine (required for memory).

When it comes to brain health, apart from making ATP, Vitamin B12 is particularly important. B12 is involved in:

- regulatory mechanisms in the brain

- the formation of blood

- DNA synthesis and regulation

- fatty acid synthesis
- the production of SAMe which is then involved in the production of neuro-transmitters, catecholaimines (dopamine, norephinephrine) and in brain metabolism.

See: http://en.wikipedia.org/wiki/Vitamin_B12

Symptoms of deficiency in B12 include:

- Depression
- Memory problems
- Mania
- Psychosis
- Brain atrophy (associated with different dementias, including Alzheimers)
- Impaired cognitive functioning
- Increased homocysteine

Like various other nutrients, one can see that a lack of B Vitamins can lead also to depression.

TWELVE

Deficiencies in Fatty Acids and Depression

We have been taught to think of the fats as bad because they cause bad cholesterols, arterio-sclerosis, obesity, diabetes, etc. But in fact, like so many medical/nutritional beliefs, this one is based on myths and misconceptions.

Your brain is made up of approximately 70% fats! So if someone calls you a fat head you can take it as a compliment.

Your brain requires very specialized kinds of fats, i.e. ALA (alpha linolenic acid – Omega 3) and LA (linoleic acid – Omega 6). From these two fatty acids you can make the longer chained DHA (docosahexaenoic acid) and AA (arachidonic acid).

With sufficient fatty acids our brain can grow and we can learn. With insufficient fatty acids – due to:

- Stress
- Poor diet
- Lack of glutathione

- Lack of vitamins and minerals
- Excess sugars/flours/potatoes
- Oxidative stress and inflammation
- Infections

We can suffer everything from cognitive distortions, emotional disorders and the inability to learn and grow.

The membranes of neurons, just like the membranes of all cells, are structured with fats. Neurons have an insulative layer around them called myelin. This myelin is about 30% protein and 70% fats. One of the most common fatty acids in myelin is oleic acid, which is found in avocados, olive oil, and a product called Xocai™ chocolate.

Unfortunately, when we intake trans fatty acids they not only get into mother's milk but then also compose part of the myelin structure wherein they change the electrical conductivity of the cells. This is very detrimental to neural functioning. Furthermore, if the body is deficient in Omega 3 ALA (alpha-linolenic acid) trans fats are doubly absorbed at the expense of Omega 3s and 6s.

However, even the balance between Omega 3s and Omega 6s are important in depression. Studies have found that diets high in Omega 6s have a positive correlation with cognitive impairment whereas diets high in Omega 3s have an inverse correlation with cognitive impairment. This imbalance can also lead to:

- Depression
- Poor Memory
- Mood swings
- Hyperactivity
- Brain allergies
- Schizophrenia

The balance of Omega 3 to 6 fatty acids influences different neurotransmitter pathways; secretion of different neurotransmitters; as well as, inflammatory/anti-inflammatory pathways. Research has indicated that omega 3 fatty acids should be utilized in various psychiatric disorders.

See:
http://www.ncbi.nlm.nih.gov/pubmed/12728744

DHA is the most abundant fat in the brain and with its deficiency comes a lack of both structural and functional capacity. A simple lack in glutathione can cause a loss of DHA which is associated with a decrease in cognitive capacity and emotional disorders.

Research has associated the increase in depression, over the last several decades, with a lack of DHA in our diets in North America. Whereas, in cultures where good fats are consumed in larger quantities show significantly less depression. Joseph R. Hibbeln, M.D., and Norman Salem, Jr., Ph.D., concluded in 1995 that the "relative deficiencies in essential fatty acids may also intensify vulnerability to depression". So this is not something new but rather, something that is just not utilized as a therapeutic modality.

DHA (docosahexaenoic acid) and AA (arachidonic acid) are very important in the development of the both the brain and the eyes and both pre- and post-natally. In fact, it has been found that infants with higher levels of DHA and AA in their diets have higher levels of intelligence, including:

- Mental Development Index
- Memory
- Ability to solve problems
- Language capacity

So, once again, we find that deficiencies in nutrition can lead to depression and cognitive disorder.

References:
http://www.fi.edu/learn/brain/fats.html#fat
sbuild

http://www.umm.edu/altmed/articles/omeg
a-3-000316.htm

http://www.sciencedaily.com/releases/2005/
05/050525161319.htm

THIRTEEN

How to Increase Serotonin levels

We have already discussed the common belief that serotonin helps keep mood elevated. And while it may not be the sole or even the primary factor in depression, it may still play a small role.

Ways to increase serotonin in your own body included:

1. Eliminate or at least reduce the processed sugars in your diet: candy, doughnuts, pastries, sodas, etc. These foods cause a rapid spike in insulin which then promotes a release of adrenaline (which is why it gives you the perceived sense of more energy). Adrenaline interferes with the production of serotonin which is why, after the initial spurt in energy, there is a crash.

2. Tryptophan is an important amino acid required to make serotonin thus it is logical to increase tryptophan foods like red meats, fish, eggs, beans, dairy and whole grains. This is particularly important when they body is stressed

whether due to emotions, lack of sleep, or poor diet (i.e., increased sugars or carbs that quickly break down into sugars.)

3. Exercise is a great anti-depressant. It doesn't have to be long distance running, or weight training or cardio workouts that people associate with the "high" but rather activities such as walking, yoga, and Tai Chi can also perform wonders. Why? It gets the body fluids moving. When the blood and lymph are moving they are moving toxins out of the body and bringing good nutrients into the body. A study published in the journal, "Physiology & Behavior" in February 1994 found that at least part of this effect is due to the fact that exercise increases serotonin production.

4. Sunshine is enormously important and creates serotonin production. When people are prone to SADS (seasonal affective disorder syndrome) they have lower levels of free serotonin. Serotonin binds to a transporter called 5-HTT – and during darker months of the year there is elevated 5-HTT binding which is associated with lower levels of serotonin at the synapses.

See:
http://www.medicalnewstoday.com/articles/
120091.php

For more reading:

How to Balance Serotonin Levels in the Gut |
eHow.com

http://www.ehow.com/how_8696693_balanc
e-serotonin-levels-gut.html#ixzz1qWqILd7r

FOURTEEN

How to increase Glutathione Levels

As has been mentioned several times, there are no transport mechanisms to transfer glutathione into the cells so we have to find ways to provoke the cells to make it.

Different research has found different methods to do this. Dr. Robert Keller's research led him to create a formulation that has all the right nutrients, in the right ratio, just like a pancake mix.

All you have to do is take the pill (OGF) and provide the cells with the pre-made mix and they will start making glutathione. The challenge here is, if the mRNA tools are not turned on then the cells can have all the pre-made mix in the world but they won't make glutathione. So we have a problem.

Along came Dr. Joe McCord who was searching for a formula to increase super oxide dismutase (SOD), perhaps the second most important anti-oxidant in the body. In the process, he found that his five-herb formulation turns on the genetic pathways not only for

SOD but also for glutathione and catalase. In addition, it also turned on the pathways for anti-inflammatories and anti-fibrosis. Wow!

So I suggest to people that they take both of these preparations. That way you get both the genetic "tools" and the "pancake mix" and then depending on the situation, I will suggest alternating them in different ways.

When you do this you get all the benefits – anti-inflammatories, anti-fibrosis and antioxidants.

FIFTEEN

How to get all the nutrients the brain needs.

When we think about chocolate we rarely think about it as brain food. There is a lot of information that is misleading about chocolate, even the bitter or dark chocolate. So let's take a good look some of these misconceptions and truths.

The regular chocolate bought from the grocery or corner store is pasteurized. It has lost all of its nutrients then wax and high fructose corn syrup have been added along with a variety of stabilizers, preservatives, colorants, etc. These substances are bad for the liver, the heart, and the waistline!

Even "bitter" or "dark" chocolate has lost most of its nutrients. It has been "dutch pressed" and had the cocoa butter – all the omega 3s taken out – which are sold at a high price for the high-end white chocolate. In the process, this chocolate lost up to 80% of the anti-oxidants that chocolate is known for but the makers of these products have a good marketing program so none of this information gets to the consumer.

Now there is another product available called Xocai™ chocolate. Xocai™ has a special patent that protects all the anti-oxidants and Omega 3s and the rest of the nutrients found in the cocoa seeds. You see, the cocoa pod has between 10 and 60 seeds per pod. Like any fruit or vegetable, it is the seed that is the most nutrient dense. This is the case with cocoa seeds as well.

This kind of chocolate is perhaps the most nutrient dense food we know of today. There are over 300 nutrients in chocolate that are hugely beneficial to the brain. No, I'm not kidding! In Xocai™, you have 19 amino acids – all the amino acids needed to make neurotransmitters. Plus, you also get some neurotransmitters, i.e. anadamide, the blissful neurotransmitter, plus endorphins – those wonderful molecules that make you feel good. In addition, you actually get real, natural anti-depressants – the real MAOIs.

This product is the number one source of magnesium in the world today. Remember the chapter on magnesium deficiency? Here is an answer.

Do you remember the need for anti-oxidants? Well, this may not be the same as glutathione, but it has 3 times the anti-oxidants that the fresh acai berry has. (Note: When acai berry is processed into a juice it loses most of its poly-phenols/anti-oxidants.) Xocai™ has 20 times the amount of anti-oxidants of green tea. In fact, 3 pieces is equivalent to 12 servings of fruit and vegetables in your anti-oxidants alone. And it is chocolate!

Now do you remember the information in the chapter on fatty acids? Oh my goodness! Xo-cai™ has protected the Omega 3 fatty acids – all the ones that the brain needs for structure, transport, fuel, communication, etc. I believe this product is awesome and yes, this gets bet-ter. It also contains Vitamins B1, B2, B3 and B12.

Does this mean that Xocai™ will "cure" your depression? No, it doesn't. What it does mean is that it can have a big impact. It may be exact-ly what you need in a whole, non-pasteurized, non-microwaved, totally clean food or it may just be part of the solution.

It is important to mention that Xocai™ is also diabetic-friendly. (In fact Xocai™ chocolate can provide a lot of help for diabetic issues.) It helps hypertension, it is good for dental hy-giene and it is great for weight loss. Can you believe it?

SIXTEEN

Exercise and Psychotherapy

When people are suffering from reactive depression, most will get better because of the passage of time, fortunate events, or positive changes in their life style.

Medications, however, can prevent people from making necessary changes in their life. European research reveals that many people who stay on antidepressants for ten years are generally worse off than those who chose healthy alternatives. Psychotherapy and exercise can help create a better life.

During all the years I practiced as just a Registered Psychologist, I always implemented exercise into my patients' recovery programs. It may be that right now you can only make it down the side walk and back but wherever you can start – start. Gradually increase how long you exercise daily. Movement will help the blood and lymph system to remove the toxins and bring fresh oxygen and nutrients to the cells, throughout the brain and through the rest of the body.

If you progress to the point that you can include activities like walking, hiking, rowing, biking, running or weight lifting so much the better. But just simply start where you currently are and keep going.

Exercise on a daily basis that involves social interaction is best. The effect of exercise is positive, both immediately and long term.

If there are additional issues like hypertension, you may want to consult a health practitioner first to see what might be the best exercise method in which to engage. Likewise, people with skeletal or muscle problems should consult with a physical therapist.

The following will be true for the vast majority of people.

- Positive psychotherapy is an effective treatment for depression (and anxiety) even if the cause began elsewhere in the body.

- Psychotherapy will be more effective and less expensive in the long run than antidepressants.

- Exercise is more effective than antidepressants.

- Treating the whole body is always the best method.

Sustaining Motion

Often a huge problem for people with passive depression (versus agitated depression) is to keep exercising. Depending on the experience of depression, some people are more likely to continue exercise if their activity involves positive social experience whereas some may prefer to start alone. Schedule times for exercise with others or if that's not possible you may even exercise just for yourself if you have the self-discipline. Exercise, healthy food and supplement, and positive psychotherapy can eliminate depression and bring joy back into your life.

Here's to your HEALTH – on all LEVELS of LIFE!